ANNA PATEL

Don't Ignore the GUT

Ultimate guide to have healthy Gut. Do's and Don'ts

This book was professionally typeset on Reedsy.
Find out more at reedsy.com

Contents

1 Introduction   1

2 CHAPTER 1 : STRUCTURE OF YOUR GUT   4

3 CHAPTER 2 : What happens to food in Gut?   6

4 CHAPTER 3 : GUT BACTERIA (GOOD vs BAD)   9

5 CHAPTER 4: WHAT CAUSES OBESITY?   15

6 CHAPTER 5: Why do I feel sleepy after eating a whole large...   20

7 CHAPTER 6: GUT CAN KILL US? GUT HEALTH vs DISEASES   27

8 CHAPTER 8: SUGAR MIGHT BE END OF US?   33

9 CHAPTER 9: HYDRATING THE GUT   36

10 CHAPTER 10: FASTING?   39

11 CHAPTER 11: MORNING FEAST   42

12 CHAPTER 12: Does exercising improve gut health?   45

13 CHAPTER 13: KEEP GUT CLEAN   49

14 BONUS: RECIPES FOR THE DAY YOU ARE FEEL-ING SICK   52

15 CONCLUSION: 55

16 REFERENCES   56

17 GRATITUDE   59

1

Introduction

If you are reading this book today then you are at the right place. I am so proud of you that you took some time out of your really busy day for your gut health. By the way, you might be wondering who I am? Well I am a first year college student, and I was too much concerned about my gut health just like you are. Why am I writing this book in the first place? So, to answer this I would like to tell you a very long story.

This is about me and my Gut. When I was very young I always had this problem of obesity. Sometimes, my stomach used to be filled with gas and I looked like a pig (no offence BTW). I wanted to be slim and fit just like that girl in my class and win my crush over her. Obesity was not my only problem, I had huge acne on my face and I always blamed it on my genetics which at some point made sense. Then one day out of nowhere, I searched this term called "Gut health" on google after watching that youtube influencer talking about taking probiotics everyday (I was curious). The moment I searched that term, Google baba showed me tons and tons of information on different boring black and white pages. I had no clue where to begin with but I was so dedicated to cure my obesity and seduce my crush so I started to look through all of those pages and sucked in all the information about Gut.

This made me realise that gut is something so important and we should never ever make the mistake of ignoring it. If you did in the past then it's completely alright because according to some great person, "It's better to be late than to arrive ugly" and "It's never too late to be what you might have been". One more thing that was stuck on my head like a chewing gum, was how can I make people aware about it. Certainly there are millions of smart people out there who know about this, but why are they still eating cookies for breakfast? Well the answer is they are just like me.

I wanted to write this book with a boring cover page, so that people will read about this and take action and be a lifesaver for their gut. I wanted to give all the information in this book in a fun way (obviously) so that you don't have to go and read those thousands of black and white pages on gut health.

So, are you ready to suck in all the information about your gut and be your own lifesaver by preventing yourselves from some nasty gut diseases. To start with, we will be going through what gut health is? Why Gut Health in the first place? And finally how to take care of it?

In these sections, there will be a lot of talk about things that can impact your gut health and how dangerous sugar is? I might also give you some skincare tips on the way so be ready for it. As there is a lot to know, you should take time to digest all the information. Emphasis is on "digest". We will also discuss some foods that we must eat to keep our gut healthy and foods that should never be consumed even if you break up with your girlfriend/ boyfriend. In addition, I will also tell you about some habits that we should avoid to have a healthy gut space. In the very beginning, we will take a quick look at some bacterias that are vital for your gut and what they are doing inside your gut twenty-four-seven (sounds creepy right).

Then we will take a sharp turn towards the reason why some people eat so much but never get fat because such people make me so jealous of them and I also envy their gut because it's the hero of the whole movie. To not make this even longer, let's begin this journey of knowing your gut.

Don't worry, I will try to not make this too boring for you so stay till the very end with me. Sometimes, things are meant to be boring so bare with me. Please. Thanks.

2

CHAPTER 1 : STRUCTURE OF YOUR GUT

For this part, I don't want to go into too much detail but I only want to touch on the topics that are important for you to know. So, the gut, which is also called the gastrointestinal tract, starts at the mouth and ends at the anus.

To break the structure down more nicely, let's talk about different parts one by one. First is our mouths. Mouth is the place where digestion begins. Next is Esophagus which we can also call a food pipe. As the name suggests, it carries food from mouth to stomach for future digestion.

In more sophisticated language, it is a muscular tube that moves food from the mouth to the stomach using rhythmic contractions called peristalsis. Further down is the stomach which is a stretchy, muscular sac that mixes food with digestive juices. The stomach breaks down food into a liquid mixture called chyme. In simple words, the stomach stores food and grinds it until it's ready to be sent to another organ. After the stomach, there is the most important organ of the gut which is called the small intestine.

It is important because it's the place where all the good things happen. Duodenum is the first part where digestive juices from the pancreas and liver mix with the chyme. Very next is Jejunum which is the middle part where nutrients are absorbed into the bloodstream. At the last is Ileum that continues nutrient absorption and passes the remaining food residue to the large intestine.

After that, we have this companion of the small intestine called large intestine or colon which is a wider tube that absorbs water and salts from the undigested food, turning it into solid waste which is called stool. It also has several parts. Cecum is the beginning part connected to the small intestine. Then, Ascending, Transverse, Descending, and Sigmoid Colon are the different sections that process waste and Rectum is the final section where stool is stored before being expelled.

Last but not the least, is the Anus. It is the opening at the end of the digestive tract where stool leaves the body.

The gut also contains various muscles and nerves that help move food along and ensure proper digestion and absorption. Additionally, it houses millions of beneficial bacteria that aid in digestion and support overall health. Yes, the bacterias that I was creeped out upon plays a very important role inside our gut and we should eat foods that help them develop more in our gut.

I hope all this information gives you a quick idea of how our gut is shaped. I will try to tell you more about this in the later chapters but for now let's move on and talk about how the food that we eat travels through the gut and what exactly happens to it.

3

CHAPTER 2 : What happens to food in Gut?

S o, as we all know, digestion starts in the mouth. You chew food, breaking it into smaller pieces. Saliva mixes with the food, beginning to break it down. The key point here is chewing. As per Ayurveda, it's the golden rule that we should chew food 32 times before swallowing it. This not only helps you to eat slowly and makes you mindful of your eating, but also helps you cope with problems like bloating, gas and other forms of indigestion problems. So, always remember to eat slowly by chewing properly.

Chewing also ensures that the food is properly mixed with our saliva because saliva which is produced by salivary gland in mouth, helps to moisten the food particle which future helps in swallowing, kill germs, neutralises some acidic foods and has proteins and minerals which protect tooth enamel. If you are someone with a dry mouth, then this is some tips for you. Drink a lot of water, chew sugar-free gums and suck on sugar-free candies. Also, eat in small amounts to ensure that you don't choke on food and this also helps in digesting the food properly.

The food then is carried to the stomach by Esophagus. Inside the stomach, the food is broken down into simpler form by the use of some digestive juices such as HCL (hydrochloric acid), pepsinogen which basically breaks the protein down into its less complex form, Gastric Lipase which is the enzyme that helps break down fats into smaller molecules. The stomach lining secretes some super mucus to protect itself from being damaged by the acidic environment. All these stomach liquids work together to ensure that food is properly broken down and prepared for further digestion and absorption in the small intestine.

From here, the food moves down to the small intestines and the climax of the movie lies here. Small intestine also releases some juices and organs like liver secretes bile juice which is all collected inside the small intestine. The inner lining of the small intestine has nodules which kind of look like hairs. These nodules are responsible to absorb the nutrients like vitamins, minerals, carbohydrates, fats, proteins from the digested food which is then used to create energy for you to do all the work. About 90% of absorption of nutrients takes place into the small intestine.

So, let's talk a little more about bacterias now. So here I am not talking about any random bacterias as the ones that are present in our gut are really good ones. Although, there are some bad bacterias too. So, what exactly does this bacterias do? Well we can say that these bacterias are in a mutual relationship with our intestine like a friends with benefits situation. So, these good bacterias help the intestine to digest food and in return they feed on some byproducts of digestion which are necessary for their survival. We will look at these byproducts in more detail in further chapters so till then hold on tight.

As we are talking about food here, I would like to add that the food that we are eating everyday is really important in a sense that it decides the amount of good or bad bacterias in our intestines. Some foods help promote the growth of good bacterias whereas others lead to formation of bad bacterias which can cause some gut health issues. Into upcoming chapters, I wanted to describe more on how different foods that we eat affect our inner body health, especially gut health. In addition to that, we are going to see what are some foods that can boost our gut health when consumed in the morning, that is, empty stomach. Foods also decide the amount of energy we get everyday. Some people feel lethargic and weak even after having a filling lunch or dinner. The reason behind this is to not intake some required nutrients that give us that energy to start our day. Majority of people suffer from gut issues due to poor eating habits. Thus, changing the way we eat is essential in maintaining a healthy gut, body and mind. Also, if the gut is not healthy then we might face problems such as acne, irregular periods in females, hormonal imbalance and many other issues that you will get to know more about as you read further.

4

CHAPTER 3 : GUT BACTERIA (GOOD vs BAD)

As I already said in the previous chapter, our intestine consists of millions and billions of bacterias which helps in digesting the food which further ensures a healthy body. I cannot name all the bacterias because it will take me more than this life to do that. So, for now let's just call those creatures in our intestines as bacterias.

In the vast and intricate world of the human body, the gut stands out as a bustling metropolis, home to trillions of microorganisms collectively known as the gut microbiota. These tiny inhabitants play a crucial role in our overall health, affecting everything from digestion and immunity to mood and metabolism. The gut microbiota is a complex community, composed of both beneficial (good) bacteria and potentially harmful (bad) bacteria. Understanding the balance between these two groups is essential for maintaining a healthy gut and, consequently, a healthy body.

Good bacteria, also known as probiotics, are the beneficial microorganisms that help keep our digestive system functioning smoothly.

They perform a variety of essential tasks. Good bacteria help break down food components that our own bodies can't digest, such as certain fibres and complex carbohydrates. This process produces short-chain fatty acids (SCFAs), which are vital for colon health and provide energy to the cells lining the gut. Probiotics (good bacterias) enhance the absorption of nutrients, including vitamins (like B vitamins and vitamin K), minerals, and amino acids, ensuring our bodies get the maximum benefit from the food we eat. It also plays a crucial role in training and modulating the immune system. They help the body distinguish between harmful pathogens and benign substances, reducing the risk of allergies and autoimmune diseases. In simple words, it strengthens your body's ability to fight the harmful virus or other pathogens that enter the body. Probiotics compete with harmful bacteria for nutrients and attachment sites on the gut lining. They also produce substances like bacteriocins and lactic acid, which inhibit the growth of bad bacteria. Emerging research suggests that good bacteria influence the gut-brain axis, affecting mood and cognitive function. Probiotics produce neurotransmitters like serotonin, which can impact mental health and well-being. Therefore, we need to take care of our gut to ensure proper mental functioning.

Let's look at some species of good bacterias. First one is, This genus includes many species that produce lactic acid, which helps maintain an acidic environment in the gut, deterring harmful bacteria. Lactobacillus is often found in fermented foods like yoghurt, kefir, and sauerkraut. Thus including these foods in daily life can help promote the growth of lactobacillus bacteria. There are other several benefits that this bacteria offers. Let's look right into it. According to several sources, it may help reduce cholesterol. Lactobacillus is effective in preventing and treating various types of diarrhea, including those caused by infections, antibiotics, and travel. By producing anti-inflammatory substances,

Lactobacillus can help reduce inflammation in the gut, which is beneficial for conditions like inflammatory bowel disease (IBD) and irritable bowel syndrome (IBS). In women, Lactobacillus helps maintain a healthy vaginal microbiota by producing lactic acid, which keeps the vaginal environment slightly acidic and prevents the overgrowth of harmful bacteria and yeast. Some studies indicate that Lactobacillus can help in weight management by influencing fat metabolism, reducing body fat, and helping regulate appetite. So, get that yoghourt bowl and eat that while you are reading this book further.

Another type of bacteria that is found in our intestine is Bifidobacterium. These bacteria are abundant in the colon and are known for their ability to break down complex carbohydrates and fibers. Bifidobacterium species are also prevalent in fermented foods and probiotic supplements. It can be found in foods such as milk kefir, sourdough bread, sauerkraut, kimchi and other fermented vegetables. I personally love kimchi as I am a rice eater and kimchi just goes so well with rice. So, next time you are having rice try having kimchi with it because it does wonders to your gut. Just like Lactobacillus, it improves the body's immune system, improves digestive health, enhances immune function, reduces inflammation, enhances nutrient absorption and reduces symptoms of lactose Intolerance. If you cannot intake dairy products like yoghurt, then this bacteria is of great help to your gut. Bifidobacterium can help digest lactose, the sugar in milk, reducing symptoms of lactose intolerance such as bloating, gas, and diarrhea.

The last bacteria that I would like to talk about is Faecalibacterium prausnitzii. Anyone would like to try speaking it five times in a row. So, this species is one of the most abundant in the human gut and is known for producing butyrate, an SCFA that supports colon health and has anti-inflammatory properties. It's fine if you don't get the complex words as the key is that this is a good bacteria and we should eat foods that don't kill it. This bacteria has Anti-Inflammatory effects and it also strengthens the gut barrier by enhancing the production of mucus and promoting the health of the gut lining. This helps prevent harmful substances from leaking into the bloodstream, reducing the risk of leaky gut syndrome. In addition, it provides energy to the cells lining the colon. This supports overall colonic health and can help prevent colon-related diseases.

Now let's see what bad bacterias are and how exactly they harm us.

Bad bacteria, or pathogenic bacteria, can disrupt the balance of the gut microbiota and contribute to various health issues. These harmful microorganisms can enter the gut through contaminated food, water, or other environmental sources. Pathogenic bacteria can cause infections in the gut, leading to conditions like gastroenteritis, food poisoning, and traveler's diarrhea. Bad bacteria can trigger inflammation in the gut, contributing to inflammatory bowel diseases (IBD) like Crohn's disease and ulcerative colitis. Chronic inflammation is also linked to other health problems, including metabolic disorders and even cancer. An overgrowth of harmful bacteria can lead to dysbiosis, an imbalance in the gut microbiota. Dysbiosis is associated with a range of conditions, from irritable bowel syndrome (IBS) and obesity to allergies and autoimmune diseases. Some bad bacteria produce toxins that damage the gut lining and disrupt normal cellular functions. For example, Clostridium difficile (C. difficile) produces toxins that can cause severe colitis, a life-threatening condition.

To prevent such bad bacteria from entering our body we need to take a close look at our eating and drinking habits. How to balance these good and bad bacterias?

Maintaining a healthy balance between good and bad bacteria is crucial for gut health. A diet rich in fiber, fruits, vegetables, and fermented foods supports the growth of good bacteria. Prebiotics, found in foods like garlic, onions, and bananas, serve as food for probiotics, helping them thrive. Probiotic supplements can help increase the population of beneficial bacteria, especially after antibiotic treatment, which can disrupt the gut microbiota. Chronic stress can negatively impact the gut microbiota. Practices like meditation, exercise, and adequate sleep can help maintain a healthy balance. So, take less stress. While antibiotics are essential for treating bacterial infections, overuse can kill both good and bad bacteria, leading to dysbiosis. It's important to use antibiotics only when necessary and under medical supervision. Never take antibiotics without a doctor's prescription as it can be really harmful to our body. Drinking plenty of water supports overall digestive health and helps maintain the mucosal lining of the intestines, where many good bacteria reside. So, stay hydrated by drinking sufficient water.

Research on the gut microbiota is rapidly evolving, revealing new insights into how these microorganisms influence our health. Future therapies may include personalized probiotics tailored to an individual's unique microbiota, fecal microbiota transplants for treating severe dysbiosis, and advanced dietary interventions to promote gut health.

In conclusion, the gut microbiota is a dynamic and complex ecosystem where good and bad bacteria coexist. Striking a balance between these microorganisms is essential for maintaining digestive health, supporting the immune system, and enhancing overall well-being. By nurturing our gut with a healthy lifestyle and mindful choices, we can ensure that the good bacteria thrive and keep the bad bacteria in check, leading to a healthier and happier life.

Before reading further I would ask you to go and drink one glass of water.
Cheers to gut health!!

5

CHAPTER 4: WHAT CAUSES OBESITY?

Obesity is excessive weight accumulation which presents a risk to health. When body mass index is over 30 then the person is called obese.

Why are we talking about obesity in the first place?

Because millions of people in the world today are stressed due to obesity and I did too at some point. Obesity can cause several other health problems to the body. Let me tell you about some health risks posed by obesity. It affects nearly all the body parts.

Obesity is a major risk factor for cardiovascular diseases, including hypertension (high blood pressure), coronary artery disease, heart attack, and stroke. Excess body fat, particularly around the abdomen, can contribute to high blood pressure by increasing the workload on the heart and promoting the buildup of plaques in the arteries (atherosclerosis). These plaques can narrow and harden the arteries, restricting blood flow and leading to heart disease and stroke.

There is a strong link between obesity and the development of type 2 diabetes. Excess fat, especially visceral fat around the abdominal organs, can cause the body's cells to become resistant to insulin, the hormone that regulates blood sugar. As a result, blood sugar levels rise, leading to insulin resistance and, eventually, type 2 diabetes. Managing obesity through weight loss can significantly reduce the risk of developing diabetes and improve blood sugar control in those already diagnosed.

Obesity is associated with an increased risk of several types of cancer, including breast, colorectal, endometrial, kidney, liver, and pancreatic cancers. The exact mechanisms are complex and multifactorial, involving factors such as chronic inflammation, hormonal imbalances (like increased estrogen levels in postmenopausal women), and insulin resistance. Fat cells produce adipokines, hormones that can promote cell proliferation and inhibit cell death, potentially leading to cancer development.

Obesity can also impair respiratory function and is a significant risk factor for obstructive sleep apnea (OSA), a condition where the airway becomes blocked during sleep, causing interrupted breathing. Excess weight, particularly around the neck, can contribute to airway obstruction. Obesity also reduces lung volume and can lead to obesity hypoventilation syndrome (OHS), where poor breathing results in low oxygen and high carbon dioxide levels in the blood.

Carrying excess weight puts additional strain on the musculoskeletal system, leading to conditions such as osteoarthritis, particularly in weight-bearing joints like the knees and hips. This added pressure accelerates the wear and tear of joint cartilage, causing pain and mobility issues. Obesity is also linked to lower back pain and can contribute to spinal disc degeneration. This is more common in grandpa's and grandma's.

Obesity increases the risk of non-alcoholic fatty liver disease (NAFLD), a condition where fat builds up in the liver, leading to inflammation and damage. NAFLD can progress to more severe liver conditions, including non-alcoholic steatohepatitis (NASH), cirrhosis, and liver failure. The prevalence of NAFLD is rising in parallel with the obesity epidemic.

Obesity can affect reproductive health in both men and women. In women, it is associated with menstrual irregularities, polycystic ovary syndrome (PCOS), and reduced fertility. In men, obesity can lead to lower testosterone levels, decreased sperm quality, and erectile dysfunction.

In addition, obesity can also cause mental and social problems. When I was a obese. I just hated to leave my house and go to school because I just did not like the way my body looked. Gradually I became so insecure of myself which led to significant decrease in my confidence and my social life was completely messed up. So, I decided to change my life not just for the sake of my social and mental health but for my body to be healthy and fit.

What food causes obesity?

I would like to give you a detailed list of all the foods that we should avoid having on weekdays. Why weekdays? Because weekends are cheat days, so it is fine to have these in limit on weekends. But always remember "too much of anything is always bad". Here are some foods to avoid:

1. Firstly, foods high in added sugars, such as candies, pastries, cakes, and sugary cereals, are dense in calories but low in nutritional value. Sugary beverages, including sodas, fruit juices, and energy drinks, are particularly problematic because they provide a large number of calories without inducing satiety, leading to increased overall

calorie intake.

2. Processed foods, including fast food items like burgers, fries, pizza, and fried chicken, are typically high in unhealthy fats, sugars, and salt. These foods are often calorie-dense and designed to be palatable and convenient, making it easy to overconsume them. Fast food also tends to be low in fiber and essential nutrients, contributing to poor diet quality.

3. Refined carbohydrates, such as white bread, white rice, pasta, and many baked goods, have had most of their fiber and nutrients removed during processing. These foods cause rapid spikes in blood sugar and insulin levels, which can lead to increased hunger and subsequent overeating. Consistently consuming refined carbs can contribute to weight gain and insulin resistance.

4. Foods high in unhealthy fats, particularly trans fats and saturated fats, can contribute to obesity. These include items like commercially baked goods, margarine, snack foods, and fried foods. While fats are a necessary part of a healthy diet, the type and amount of fat consumed are crucial. Healthy fats, such as those found in avocados, nuts, and olive oil, should be preferred over unhealthy options.

5. Snack foods like chips, crackers, cookies, and granola bars are often high in calories, unhealthy fats, sugars, and salt. These convenient, packaged foods are designed to be highly palatable and easy to overeat. They also tend to have little to no nutritional value, contributing to excessive calorie intake without providing essential nutrients.

6. Alcoholic beverages are calorie-dense and can contribute significantly to daily calorie intake. Additionally, alcohol can lower inhibitions and increase appetite, leading to overeating. High-calorie alcoholic beverages, such as cocktails made with sugary mixers, are particularly likely to contribute to weight gain.

7. Consuming large portions of any type of food can lead to excessive calorie intake. Restaurant meals, particularly in fast food and casual dining establishments, often feature oversized portions that can significantly exceed caloric needs. Additionally, the practice of "supersizing" meals can further exacerbate this issue.

8. Condiments and sauces, such as mayonnaise, creamy dressings, and sugary sauces, can add a significant number of calories to meals without providing substantial nutritional benefits. These additions can easily lead to an excess caloric intake, contributing to weight gain.

I know you might be thinking what am I supposed to eat when 70% of things are something that I should avoid. Well I had the same question when I was in your shoes. But don't worry I won't leave you starving. I would try to give you some tips on how to make boring healthy food tasty.

Now let's talk about energy a bit. So, when I was a student I always faced this problem of feeling lethargic and sleepy all day. This was because I liked eating foods that I have mentioned above which certainly did not give me energy to function for the whole day. This was affecting my daily activities and especially my studies.

I decided to make a whole chapter on this so all feel energetic in future. On that saying, it's time for your next glass of water. If you are not feeling very thirsty then just drink a bit. Cheers on energy!

6

CHAPTER 5: Why do I feel sleepy after eating a whole large sized Pizza?

re you one of those people who feels sleepy after a huge meal? If you are not then let me tell you that I can sleep for five hours right after eating a huge cheese pizza. So, don't worry this is not something abnormal. Feeling sleepy after eating might be a natural result of digestion and sleep patterns. It depends upon what kind of food we are eating. According to researchers, feeling tired after eating is something natural and common amongst people and it usually does not require any concern. In scientific language, a decrease in energy levels after eating is called postprandial somnolence.

Is it good to sleep right after eating a heavy meal?

So, the answer is a complete **NO**. We need to wait for about three hours after eating to sleep. Going to bed right after eating a huge cheese pizza can cause certain problems like poor sleep, slower metabolism, acid reflux, indigestion and heartburn. If your are someone who faces problems such as acidity, gas or bloating after sleep then it might be because you are not giving time to your food to digest before laying down to sleep. Additionally, several studies show that eating at late night can be less filling and can cause more calorie intake and calories are the worst enemy of gut. So, let's try and control those late night cravings because they are bad for the gut.

Sleeping after a heavy meal can also lead to unnecessary weight gain. As per the facts, this might be due to metabolism and insulin. Therefore, we should not sleep right after eating.

What foods can make you feel tired or sleepy?

Certain foods are more likely to make you feel tired after eating, a phenomenon influenced by several factors including the food's composition and its effects on your body's physiology. One primary reason is the macronutrient composition of the meal, particularly the balance of carbohydrates, proteins, and fats. So, eating a meal that is balanced is very important.

Foods high in carbohydrates, especially those rich in simple sugars and refined grains, can lead to a rapid spike in blood sugar levels. This spike is often followed by a swift drop, which can result in feelings of fatigue. Common examples include sweets, white bread, pasta, and other processed foods. The body releases insulin to manage the sudden influx of sugar, and this process can cause an overcorrection, leading to low blood sugar and subsequent tiredness.

In addition to carbohydrates, foods rich in tryptophan, an amino acid found in protein-rich foods like turkey, chicken, dairy products, and nuts, can also make you feel sleepy. Tryptophan is a precursor to serotonin, a neurotransmitter that plays a role in sleep regulation. When consumed in large amounts, tryptophan can increase the production of serotonin and subsequently melatonin, a hormone that promotes sleep, thereby making you feel drowsy.

Meals high in fat can also contribute to post-meal drowsiness. Fatty foods take longer to digest, and the process requires a significant amount of energy. As your body diverts blood flow to the digestive system to manage this heavy workload, you may experience a drop in overall energy levels, leading to fatigue. Examples of such foods include fried items, creamy sauces, and fatty cuts of meat.

Another factor is the overall size of the meal. Large, heavy meals can lead to a condition known as postprandial somnolence, commonly referred to as a "food coma." This is because a large meal requires more digestive effort, increasing blood flow to the stomach and intestines and reducing the blood flow available to the rest of the body, including the brain, thus causing feelings of tiredness.

In summary, foods high in simple carbohydrates, tryptophan-rich proteins, and fats can make you feel tired due to their effects on blood sugar levels, serotonin production, and the digestive workload. Additionally, the sheer volume of food consumed in a single sitting can exacerbate these effects, leading to significant post-meal drowsiness.

I want to describe more on what happens when we sleep right after eating such foods.

Sleeping after eating foods that induce tiredness can have several effects on your body and overall health, both positive and negative.

When you lie down soon after eating, digestion can be less efficient. Gravity helps food move through your digestive system, and lying down can disrupt this process, potentially leading to indigestion or heartburn, especially if you've eaten a large or fatty meal.

Lying down can increase the risk of acid reflux or gastroesophageal reflux disease (GERD). This is because the position can allow stomach acid to move back up into the esophagus more easily.

It can also affect the quality of sleep. Eating a heavy meal before bed can interfere with your sleep cycles. While you might fall asleep quickly due to the production of serotonin and melatonin, the body's active digestion process can disrupt sleep later in the night, leading to fragmented sleep and frequent awakenings. There is anecdotal evidence suggesting that eating certain foods, particularly those high in sugar or spicy foods, before bed can lead to more vivid dreams or even nightmares. This is thought to be related to increased metabolic activity and brain waves during digestion. I don't know if this is true or not but it is an interesting topic to do some more research. It might be a myth though. Have you ever experienced this?

Apart from that, consuming foods high in sugar or refined carbohydrates can cause a spike in insulin levels, which can be followed by a drop in blood sugar. This fluctuation might not only make you feel sleepy initially but can also lead to waking up in the middle of the night if your blood sugar drops too low. Late-night eating, particularly of high-calorie, high-fat foods, can contribute to weight gain. The body's metabolism slows down during sleep, so excess calories consumed before bedtime are more likely to be stored as fat.

What are some practices to follow to avoid such practice?

- Eat Smaller Meals: Try to eat smaller, more balanced meals that include a mix of carbohydrates, proteins, and fats.
- Timing: Allow at least 2-3 hours between eating and going to bed to give your body enough time to begin digesting the food.
- Avoid Trigger Foods: Steer clear of foods known to cause heartburn or indigestion, such as spicy foods, high-fat meals, and caffeine.
- Stay Upright: Stay upright after eating, perhaps by taking a light walk, to help with digestion and prevent reflux.

And, be mindful of what you are eating. I know it is not that easy but trust me once you start it and keep doing it for twenty-one days it won't be that hard anymore as the body and mind will adapt to it. By doing this you can improve your sleep and digestion.

What kind of foods or drinks are good to consume at late night?

If you are someone who cannot cut on their late night cravings then let me give you some recommendations on foods that you can eat before sleep and might help with your sleep. If you are allergic to any of these foods then I advise you not to consume it. Ask for your nutritionist's advice because they definitely know more.

Here are some recommendations:

1. Complex Carbohydrates:

- Whole Grain Crackers: Whole grain options provide fiber and steady energy release without causing blood sugar spikes.
- Oatmeal: A small bowl of oatmeal is filling and can promote the production of melatonin, a sleep-regulating hormone.

1. Lean Proteins:

- Turkey: Contains tryptophan, which can help induce sleep.
- Greek Yogurt: High in protein and contains calcium, which helps the brain use tryptophan to produce melatonin.

1. Fruits and Vegetables:

- Bananas: Rich in potassium and magnesium, which help relax muscles.
- Cherries: Natural source of melatonin.
- Kiwifruit: Studies suggest it may improve sleep quality due to its high serotonin content.

1. Nuts and Seeds:

- Almonds: Provide magnesium, which is good for muscle relaxation and sleep.
- Pumpkin Seeds: Contain magnesium and tryptophan.

1. Dairy:

- Warm Milk: Contains tryptophan and has a soothing effect that can promote sleep.

Drinks

1. Herbal Teas:

- Chamomile Tea: Known for its calming properties and can help improve sleep quality.
- Peppermint Tea: Helps with digestion and has a soothing effect on the stomach.
- Lavender Tea: Has mild sedative effects and promotes relaxation.

1. Golden Milk:

- Turmeric Latte: Made with milk and turmeric, which has anti-inflammatory properties and promotes relaxation.

General Tips:

- Moderation: Keep portions small to avoid overloading your digestive system.
- Avoid High Sugar and Fat: Foods and drinks high in sugar and fat

can cause energy spikes and digestive issues, disrupting sleep.
- Stay Hydrated: Drink enough water, but avoid excessive fluids that might cause you to wake up for bathroom trips.

Sample Late-Night Snack Ideas:

- A small bowl of oatmeal with a few slices of banana and a sprinkle of almonds.
- A handful of cherries or a kiwi.
- Whole grain crackers with a small serving of low-fat cheese.
- A cup of chamomile tea with a teaspoon of honey.
- Greek yogurt topped with a few pumpkin seeds.

I found all these on the internet and I have tried them but if something does not suit your body then please avoid it. I hope you liked these recommendations and feel free to try them but be careful of allergies.

Good job to reach till here. Now you know a lot about gut. If I am wrong then my apologies. By the way, don't forget to hydrate your body today. Cheers to good health and sleep!!

7

CHAPTER 6: GUT CAN KILL US? GUT HEALTH vs DISEASES

Gut health is very important because it absorbs the food we eat by breaking it down and supports our body to perform daily functions. Poor gut health can cause several problems in our later life stages. For teenagers and young adults, having a healthy gut is very important.

What factors affect gut health negatively ?

Stress, insomnia or lack of sleep, insufficient physical activities, imbalance in diet, eating too much processed food, smoking and drinking are all the factors that can lead to gut health issues.

Alcohol consumption, especially when excessive, can have significant adverse effects on gut health.Alcohol alters the composition of the gut microbiota, often leading to a decrease in beneficial bacteria and an increase in harmful bacteria. This imbalance, known as dysbiosis, can impair the gut's ability to function correctly and protect against pathogens.Chronic alcohol consumption can increase gut permeability, a condition often referred to as "leaky gut." This happens because alcohol damages the tight junctions between intestinal cells, allowing toxins, bacteria, and undigested food particles to enter the bloodstream. This leakage can trigger systemic inflammation and contribute to various health issues, including liver disease and autoimmune conditions.Alcohol-induced gut permeability and dysbiosis can lead to chronic inflammation. The immune system responds to the presence of foreign substances in the bloodstream, resulting in an inflammatory response. Over time, this chronic inflammation can contribute to the development of gastrointestinal diseases, such as gastritis, pancreatitis, and inflammatory bowel disease (IBD).Alcohol can interfere with the absorption of essential nutrients, such as vitamins and minerals, in the intestines. This can lead to deficiencies and related health problems. For instance, alcohol impairs the absorption of vitamin B12, folic acid, and zinc, which are crucial for maintaining overall health and proper immune function.The gut-liver axis is a critical pathway connecting gut health to liver function. Alcohol consumption can lead to liver disease through this axis. When the gut barrier is compromised, endotoxins from gut bacteria can enter the liver via the portal vein, causing inflammation and damage. This process can lead to conditions like alcoholic fatty liver disease, hepatitis, and cirrhosis.

Smoking also exerts several detrimental effects on gut health, which are well-documented in scientific literature.

Like alcohol, smoking disrupts the balance of the gut microbiota. Studies have shown that smokers have a distinct gut microbiome compared to non-smokers, characterized by a reduction in beneficial bacteria and an increase in harmful ones. This dysbiosis can contribute to various gastrointestinal disorders. Smoking is a well-established risk factor for the development of Crohn's disease, a type of inflammatory bowel disease (IBD). Smokers are more likely to develop Crohn's disease, and the disease course tends to be more severe in smokers compared to non-smokers. However, interestingly, smoking appears to have a protective effect against ulcerative colitis, another form of IBD, though the reasons for this are not fully understood. The toxins in cigarette smoke can impair the immune system's function, making the gut more susceptible to infections and inflammation. Smoking-induced immune dysregulation can exacerbate the severity of gastrointestinal diseases and impair the body's ability to respond to gut-related illnesses.Smoking affects the blood flow to the gut, impairing the healing of the intestinal lining. This can exacerbate the damage caused by conditions like peptic ulcers and contribute to the development of chronic gastrointestinal issues.

In conclusion, Both alcohol and smoking have profound and detrimental effects on gut health. They disrupt the gut microbiota, increase gut permeability, trigger inflammation, and impair the gut's ability to absorb nutrients and heal. These changes can lead to a range of gastrointestinal disorders and systemic health issues. Reducing or eliminating alcohol consumption and smoking can significantly improve gut health and overall well-being.

What are some signs of poor gut health?

Poor gut health can manifest in various ways, affecting not just the digestive system but also overall physical and mental well-being. Frequent gas, bloating, and abdominal pain are common signs that your gut is not functioning optimally. These symptoms can indicate conditions like irritable bowel syndrome (IBS) or small intestinal bacterial overgrowth (SIBO).

Persistent constipation, diarrhea, or alternating between the two can be indicative of gut dysbiosis or other gastrointestinal disorders. Experiencing regular heartburn or acid reflux might suggest that your gut is struggling to process and move food effectively.Developing intolerances or sensitivities to certain foods, such as dairy, gluten, or certain carbohydrates, can signal that your gut health is compromised. Feeling constantly tired, even after adequate rest, can be linked to poor gut health. An unhealthy gut can impact your ability to absorb nutrients and produce energy. Conditions like acne, eczema, and psoriasis can be related to gut health. Inflammation and dysbiosis in the gut can trigger skin problems.A significant portion of the immune system resides in the gut. Poor gut health can weaken the immune response, making you more susceptible to infections and illnesses.Problems with concentration, memory, and mental clarity, often referred to as "brain fog," can be associated with an unhealthy gut. Emerging research suggests that gut health is linked to autoimmune diseases. An unhealthy gut can trigger systemic inflammation and alter immune function, potentially leading to conditions like rheumatoid arthritis, lupus, and multiple sclerosis. Chronic bad breath, or halitosis, can be a sign of bacterial overgrowth in the gut or poor digestion. An imbalance in gut bacteria can lead to increased cravings for sugary foods, which can further exacerbate gut health issues.

What are some diseases caused due to poor gut?

Poor gut health can lead to a variety of diseases and conditions that affect not just the digestive system but also other parts of the body. Here are some notable diseases and conditions associated with poor gut health.

Irritable Bowel Syndrome (IBS) which can be characterized by chronic abdominal pain, bloating, and altered bowel habits (constipation, diarrhea, or both). Dysbiosis and gut motility issues are often implicated.

Inflammatory Bowel Disease (IBD) which also Includes Crohn's disease and ulcerative colitis. These conditions involve chronic inflammation of the gastrointestinal tract, which is linked to an abnormal immune response and gut microbiota imbalance.

Small Intestinal Bacterial Overgrowth (SIBO). Occurs when there is an excessive growth of bacteria in the small intestine, leading to symptoms like bloating, diarrhea, and malabsorption.

Celiac Disease is an autoimmune disorder triggered by the ingestion of gluten, leading to damage in the small intestine. Poor gut health can exacerbate symptoms and complications.

Gastroesophageal Reflux Disease (GERD) is a chronic acid reflux that can be associated with gut dysbiosis and impaired digestion.

Type 2 Diabetes, Dysbiosis is linked to insulin resistance and metabolic syndrome, contributing to the development of type 2 diabetes.

Non-Alcoholic Fatty Liver Disease (NAFLD) leads to poor gut health and increased gut permeability can lead to the translocation of endotoxins to the liver, causing inflammation and fat accumulation.

Some other autoimmune diseases are:

Rheumatoid Arthritis. Dysbiosis and leaky gut can trigger systemic inflammation and autoimmune responses, contributing to conditions like rheumatoid arthritis.

Multiple Sclerosis (MS). Emerging research suggests that gut health may play a role in the development and progression of MS due to its influence on the immune system.

As discussed earlier, it can also cause some mental health issues like depression and anxiety and Autism Spectrum Disorder (ASD), research indicates that gut microbiota imbalances may influence the development and severity of ASD symptoms.

It can also cause some skin issues like Acne, Gut dysbiosis and leaky gut can contribute to systemic inflammation, which can manifest as skin conditions like acne. Eczema and Psoriasis caused by poor gut health and an imbalanced immune response can exacerbate these inflammatory skin conditions.

Some other cardiovascular diseases are:

Atherosclerosis: Inflammation and endotoxins from a leaky gut can contribute to the development of plaque in the arteries, leading to atherosclerosis and cardiovascular diseases.

Surprisingly bad gut can also cause health risks like Asthma and Allergies. Dysbiosis and an overactive immune response due to poor gut health can increase the risk of developing allergies and asthma.

Maintaining good gut health is crucial for preventing a wide range of diseases and conditions. A balanced diet rich in fiber, probiotics, and prebiotics, along with a healthy lifestyle that includes regular exercise, adequate sleep, and stress management, can help support gut health and reduce the risk of these diseases. If you suspect gut health issues, it's important to consult with a healthcare provider for proper diagnosis and treatment.

Therefore, the gut might kill us if we don't take care of it. So, in the upcoming chapters we will look how exactly we can take care of our gut.

8

CHAPTER 8: SUGAR MIGHT BE END OF US?

"The Bittersweet Truth: Sugar's Impact on Gut Health"

In the intricate ecosystem of the human body, the gut reigns supreme as a crucial player in maintaining overall health and well-being. Comprising trillions of microorganisms, the gut microbiome influences digestion, immunity, and even mental health. However, lurking amidst the modern diet is a silent assailant: sugar. While often indulged in without much thought, sugar's insidious effects on gut health are increasingly coming to light, prompting concerns among health experts and consumers alike.

At its core, the gut microbiome is a diverse community of bacteria, viruses, fungi, and other microorganisms that reside in the gastrointestinal tract. This microbial menagerie plays a pivotal role in various physiological processes, including nutrient absorption, immune function regulation, and even mood modulation. However, the delicate balance of this ecosystem can be disrupted by dietary factors, with sugar emerging as a notorious disruptor.

The average Western diet is inundated with sugar, often in the form of refined sugars and high-fructose corn syrup added to processed foods and sugary beverages. Excessive sugar consumption not only contributes to weight gain and metabolic disorders but also exerts detrimental effects on gut health. One of the primary mechanisms through which sugar wreaks havoc on the gut is by promoting the overgrowth of harmful bacteria while suppressing beneficial strains.

Research indicates that a high-sugar diet can lead to dysbiosis, an imbalance in gut microbial composition characterized by an overabundance of pathogenic bacteria and a depletion of beneficial species. This dysbiotic state is associated with various gastrointestinal disorders, including irritable bowel syndrome (IBS), inflammatory bowel disease (IBD), and even colorectal cancer. Moreover, dysbiosis can compromise gut barrier function, leading to increased intestinal permeability, commonly referred to as "leaky gut."

Leaky gut syndrome, a condition marked by the abnormal permeability of the intestinal lining, allows harmful substances such as toxins, undigested food particles, and bacteria to leak into the bloodstream. This triggers an immune response, leading to systemic inflammation and potentially contributing to the development of chronic diseases, including autoimmune disorders and metabolic syndrome. Sugar's role in exacerbating leaky gut underscores its detrimental impact on overall health.

Furthermore, sugar consumption fuels the proliferation of pathogenic bacteria like Clostridia and Candida, which can produce toxins and inflammatory compounds, further disrupting gut homeostasis. These harmful microbes thrive on sugar, creating a vicious cycle of dysbiosis and inflammation within the gut environment. Additionally, excessive sugar intake promotes the growth of yeast species like Candida albicans, which can lead to fungal overgrowth and systemic infections in susceptible individuals.

Beyond directly influencing gut microbiota composition, sugar consumption also interferes with the production of short-chain fatty acids (SCFAs), essential compounds synthesized by beneficial gut bacteria through the fermentation of dietary fiber. SCFAs, particularly butyrate, play a crucial role in maintaining gut barrier integrity, modulating immune responses, and providing energy for colonocytes. By depriving beneficial bacteria of their primary fuel source—dietary fiber—and promoting the growth of sugar-loving pathogens, excessive sugar intake compromises SCFA production, further compromising gut health.

Addressing the detrimental impact of sugar on gut health requires a multifaceted approach, including dietary modifications and lifestyle interventions. Reducing the consumption of added sugars and opting for whole, nutrient-dense foods can help restore microbial balance and promote gut health. Additionally, incorporating dietary fiber-rich foods such as fruits, vegetables, legumes, and whole grains can support the growth of beneficial bacteria and enhance SCFA production.

In conclusion, while sugar may satisfy our sweet cravings, its toll on gut health is undeniable. From fostering dysbiosis and leaky gut syndrome to fueling inflammation and immune dysfunction, excessive sugar consumption poses a significant threat to the delicate balance of the gut microbiome. By recognizing the bittersweet truth of sugar's impact and adopting healthier dietary habits, we can nurture our gut ecosystem and safeguard our overall well-being.

9

CHAPTER 9: HYDRATING THE GUT

In the realm of wellness, hydration often takes center stage, celebrated for its myriad benefits ranging from improved skin health to enhanced physical performance. However, its significance extends far beyond quenching thirst; hydration plays a pivotal role in maintaining gut health, fostering optimal digestion, nutrient absorption, and overall well-being. Understanding the intricate relationship between hydration and gut function underscores the importance of adequate fluid intake in supporting gastrointestinal health.

The gastrointestinal tract, often referred to as the gut, is a complex system responsible for digesting food, absorbing nutrients, and eliminating waste. Comprising various organs, including the stomach, small intestine, and colon, the gut relies on a delicate balance of factors to function efficiently. Adequate hydration is essential for preserving this balance and facilitating the myriad physiological processes that occur within the digestive system.

Water serves as the primary component of digestive fluids, including saliva, gastric juices, and intestinal secretions, all of which are essential for breaking down food and facilitating nutrient absorption. Insufficient hydration can lead to decreased saliva production, impairing the initial stages of digestion and compromising oral health. Additionally, inadequate fluid intake can hinder gastric acid secretion, which is crucial for the breakdown of proteins and the activation of digestive enzymes in the stomach.

Moreover, hydration plays a vital role in maintaining the integrity of the gastrointestinal mucosa, the protective lining that lines the digestive tract. A well-hydrated mucosal barrier acts as a defense mechanism against harmful pathogens, toxins, and irritants present in food and the environment. Dehydration, on the other hand, can compromise mucosal integrity, leading to increased permeability and susceptibility to inflammation and gastrointestinal disorders.

One of the most common gastrointestinal complaints associated with dehydration is constipation. Insufficient fluid intake can result in dry, hard stools and impaired bowel motility, making it difficult to pass waste effectively. Chronic dehydration contributes to recurring constipation, which, if left unaddressed, can lead to discomfort, bloating, and more severe complications such as fecal impaction and hemorrhoids.

In addition to promoting regular bowel movements, proper hydration supports the growth and activity of beneficial gut bacteria, collectively known as the gut microbiota. These microbial inhabitants play a crucial role in maintaining gut health by fermenting dietary fiber, synthesizing vitamins, and modulating immune function. Adequate hydration ensures optimal conditions for microbial proliferation and activity, fostering a diverse and resilient gut microbiome.

Furthermore, hydration facilitates the transport of nutrients across the intestinal epithelium, ensuring efficient absorption and utilization by the body. Water acts as a solvent, aiding in the dissolution and breakdown of nutrients for absorption into the bloodstream. Without adequate hydration, nutrient absorption may be compromised, leading to deficiencies and impaired overall health.

Beyond its direct effects on gut function, hydration influences various factors that indirectly impact gastrointestinal health. Proper fluid balance supports thermoregulation, electrolyte balance, and circulation, all of which contribute to overall physiological homeostasis. Moreover, staying hydrated promotes satiety and aids in weight management, reducing the risk of obesity-related gastrointestinal conditions such as gastroesophageal reflux disease (GERD) and non-alcoholic fatty liver disease (NAFLD).

In conclusion, hydration is indispensable for maintaining gut health and supporting optimal digestive function. By ensuring adequate fluid intake, individuals can promote proper digestion, nutrient absorption, and bowel regularity while fortifying the integrity of the gastrointestinal mucosa and nurturing a diverse gut microbiome. Embracing hydration as a cornerstone of gastrointestinal wellness empowers individuals to prioritize their health and cultivate a thriving gut ecosystem.

Therefore, remember to drink sufficient water everyday. Cheers to hydrating the gut!!

10

CHAPTER 10: FASTING?

Fasting, the practice of abstaining from food and, in some cases, drink for a specified period, has been revered for centuries for its purported health benefits. Beyond its religious and cultural significance, fasting has garnered attention in recent years for its potential to promote gut health and overall well-being. While fasting regimens vary in duration and methodology, emerging research suggests that intermittent fasting and other fasting protocols may indeed confer various advantages for gut health.

Intermittent fasting (IF), characterized by alternating periods of fasting and eating, has gained popularity as a dietary strategy for weight management, metabolic health, and longevity. One of the key mechanisms through which intermittent fasting exerts its beneficial effects on gut health is by promoting autophagy, a cellular process that facilitates the removal of damaged organelles and proteins. Autophagy plays a crucial role in maintaining gut barrier integrity, reducing inflammation, and protecting against gastrointestinal disorders.

During fasting periods, cellular energy depletion triggers the activation of autophagy, enabling cells to recycle dysfunctional components and mitigate oxidative stress. In the context of gut health, autophagy helps clear away damaged epithelial cells, prevent the accumulation of toxic byproducts, and enhance the renewal of the intestinal lining. By promoting cellular cleansing and rejuvenation, intermittent fasting supports gut barrier function and resilience against environmental insults.

Moreover, intermittent fasting has been shown to modulate the composition and diversity of the gut microbiota, the community of microorganisms inhabiting the gastrointestinal tract. Research indicates that fasting regimens can promote the growth of beneficial bacteria while suppressing the proliferation of pathogenic strains. This microbial remodeling is associated with improved metabolic health, reduced inflammation, and enhanced gut barrier integrity.

Furthermore, intermittent fasting stimulates the production of short-chain fatty acids (SCFAs), microbial metabolites with potent anti-inflammatory and immunomodulatory properties. SCFAs, such as butyrate, acetate, and propionate, are generated through the fermentation of dietary fiber by gut bacteria. By promoting a fasting-induced shift towards SCFA-producing bacteria, intermittent fasting fosters a gut environment that is conducive to health and resilience.

Beyond intermittent fasting, extended fasting protocols, such as water fasting and prolonged fasting, have also been investigated for their potential gut benefits. These more prolonged fasting regimens offer a deeper state of metabolic rest, allowing for enhanced autophagy, cellular repair, and regeneration. While research on extended fasting and gut health is still evolving, preliminary evidence suggests that periodic extended fasts may promote gut rejuvenation and mitigate gastrointestinal inflammation.

However, it's essential to approach fasting with caution and individualize fasting regimens based on health status, medical history, and nutritional needs. Fasting may not be suitable for everyone, particularly individuals with certain medical conditions, such as diabetes, eating disorders, or pregnant and lactating women. Additionally, prolonged fasting without proper supervision and support can pose risks of nutrient deficiencies, electrolyte imbalances, and other adverse effects.

In conclusion, fasting holds promise as a potential strategy for promoting gut health through mechanisms such as autophagy induction, microbiota modulation, and SCFA production. Intermittent fasting, in particular, has emerged as a popular approach for harnessing these gut benefits while supporting metabolic health and longevity. However, it's crucial to approach fasting mindfully, prioritize hydration and nutrient adequacy, and seek guidance from healthcare professionals when embarking on fasting regimens. With careful consideration and moderation, fasting may offer a holistic approach to nurturing gut health and optimizing overall well-being.

In my culture, we fast almost four to five times a month and after every fasting it feels as if my gut has been completely renovated. If you don't like fasting then I would advise you to do intermittent fasting. Or else what you can do is eat only light foods for one meal and then eat nothing the whole day. This is also a type of fasting. Fasting is proven to be good for health but every person has a different body so if fasting does not suits your body type then you should avoid doing it.

11

CHAPTER 11: MORNING FEAST

The dawn of each day presents an opportunity to nourish not only our bodies but also our intricate gut microbiome, a bustling community of microorganisms that play a pivotal role in our overall health. The foods and drinks we choose to consume in the morning can set the stage for optimal digestion, nutrient absorption, and gut health throughout the day. By selecting gut-friendly options rich in fiber, probiotics, and other beneficial nutrients, we can cultivate a thriving ecosystem within our digestive tract. Incorporating probiotic foods into your morning routine introduces live beneficial bacteria to your gut, promoting microbial diversity and balance. Yogurt, kefir, and fermented vegetables like sauerkraut and kimchi are excellent sources of probiotics. These foods not only support digestion but also bolster immune function and may alleviate gastrointestinal issues such as bloating and constipation. Fruits are nature's bounty, offering a treasure trove of vitamins, minerals, antioxidants, and fiber. Opt for fiber-rich fruits like berries, apples, pears, and bananas to kickstart your day with a dose of gut-friendly nutrients. Fiber promotes bowel regularity, feeds beneficial gut bacteria, and helps maintain a healthy gut lining, reducing the risk of gastrointestinal disorders. Start your morning with whole grains like oats, quinoa, barley, or whole wheat bread for sustained energy and gut health benefits. Whole grains are rich in insoluble fiber, which adds bulk to stools and facilitates smooth bowel movements. Including whole grains in your breakfast provides a steady supply of fiber to support digestive function and promote satiety. Chia seeds and flax seeds are also great for morning breakfast as these tiny nutritional powerhouses are packed with fiber, omega-3 fatty acids, and antioxidants, making them an excellent addition to your morning routine. Sprinkle chia seeds or ground flaxseeds over yogurt, oatmeal, or smoothies to boost fiber intake, support heart health, and promote a healthy gut microbiom.

Prebiotics are non-digestible fibers that serve as fuel for beneficial gut bacteria, promoting their growth and activity. Include prebiotic-rich foods like onions, garlic, leeks, asparagus, and Jerusalem artichokes in your morning meals to support a healthy gut microbiome. These foods not only feed beneficial bacteria but also enhance nutrient absorption and immune function.

Herbal teas such as ginger, peppermint, and chamomile have long been revered for their digestive benefits. Enjoy a cup of herbal tea alongside your breakfast to soothe the digestive tract, alleviate bloating and gas, and promote overall gut health. Herbal teas provide a calming and comforting start to your day while supporting optimal digestion. I personally like to make myself a Indian spice herbal tea in the morning which include lemon, honey and ginger. Lemon is good for both skin and gut. For some people, drinking something acetic in the morning can lead to acid reflux later in the day. So, avoid it if you are that person.

If you are someone who like a meaty morning then a warm cup of bone broth in the morning can provide essential nutrients like collagen, gelatin, and amino acids that support gut lining integrity and repair. Bone broth is soothing to the digestive system and may help alleviate symptoms of gastrointestinal discomfort. Incorporating bone broth into your morning routine can nourish your gut and promote overall digestive wellness.

Incorporating these gut-friendly foods and drinks into your morning routine can help lay the foundation for a healthy gut and overall well-being. By prioritizing nutrient-rich, fiber-filled foods, probiotic-rich fermented foods, and soothing herbal teas, you can nourish your gut and support digestive wellness from the moment you wake up. Remember to listen to your body, experiment with different foods and drinks, and find what works best for you in promoting a happy and healthy gut.

Morning breakfasts are really important because it gives you energy for the rest of the day. So, never miss your morning breakfast. So, what is your favourite thing to have for breakfast? Share your recipe with your loved ones and make your morning more special and enjoyable.

12

CHAPTER 12: Does exercising improve gut health?

Exercise is renowned for its multitude of benefits, from enhancing cardiovascular health to improving mood and cognition. Yet, its impact on gut health is a lesser-known but equally significant aspect of its physiological effects. Engaging in regular physical activity can exert profound positive influences on the gut, fostering a balanced microbiome, enhancing digestive function, and mitigating gastrointestinal disorders. Here's how exercise contributes to gut health.

Regular exercise has been shown to increase microbial diversity within the gut, enriching the ecosystem with a variety of beneficial bacteria. A diverse microbiome is associated with improved digestion, stronger immunity, and reduced inflammation. Exercise-induced shifts in microbial composition have been linked to enhanced metabolic health and a lower risk of obesity and metabolic disorders.

Chronic inflammation in the gut is a hallmark of many gastrointestinal disorders, including inflammatory bowel diseases (IBD) and irritable bowel syndrome (IBS). Exercise has anti-inflammatory effects through-out the body, including the gut. Physical activity helps modulate inflam-matory cytokines, reducing gut inflammation and promoting a healthier gut environment. This may alleviate symptoms of inflammatory gut conditions and improve overall digestive well-being.

Exercise stimulates intestinal contractions and promotes peristalsis, the wave-like movement of the digestive tract that propels food and waste through the intestines. By enhancing gut motility, exercise can alleviate symptoms of constipation and promote regular bowel movements. This improved bowel function supports overall digestive health and reduces the risk of gastrointestinal discomfort and complications.

The intestinal barrier serves as a protective barrier, preventing harmful substances from entering the bloodstream while allowing the absorption of nutrients. Exercise has been shown to enhance gut barrier integrity by upregulating the expression of tight junction proteins that maintain the integrity of the intestinal lining. A robust gut barrier is crucial for preventing leaky gut syndrome and reducing systemic inflammation.Ex-ercise influences the metabolic activity of gut microbes, leading to the production of beneficial metabolites such as short-chain fatty acids (SCFAs). SCFAs play a key role in maintaining gut health by nourishing colonocytes, modulating immune responses, and regulating appetite and energy metabolism. By promoting SCFA production, exercise supports a healthy gut environment and metabolic homeostasis.

It also Alleviates Stress-Related Gut Symptoms. Stress has a profound impact on gut health, exacerbating symptoms of gastrointestinal dis-orders such as IBS and exacerbating gut inflammation. Exercise is a potent stress reliever, triggering the release of endorphins and reducing levels of stress hormones like cortisol. Regular physical activity can help alleviate stress-related gut symptoms, improve mood, and promote overall emotional well-being.Exercise increases blood flow to various organs, including the digestive system, promoting nutrient delivery and waste removal. Enhanced blood flow to the gut supports optimal digestive function, accelerates tissue repair, and contributes to overall gut health.

In conclusion, exercise is a powerful ally in the quest for optimal gut health. By promoting microbial diversity, reducing inflammation, enhancing gut motility, supporting barrier function, boosting microbial metabolism, alleviating stress-related symptoms, and improving blood flow to the gut, regular physical activity provides a comprehensive array of benefits for digestive wellness. Incorporating exercise into your daily routine, whether it's through aerobic activities, strength training, or yoga, can play a vital role in nurturing a healthy gut and promoting overall well-being.

Some yoga poses offers a holistic approach to improving gut health by combining physical postures, breathing techniques, and mindfulness practices. Certain yoga poses specifically target the digestive system, promoting digestion, relieving gastrointestinal discomfort, and fostering overall gut wellness.

Apanasana (Knee-to-Chest Pose) is a gentle yoga pose that massages the abdomen, stimulates digestion, and relieves bloating and gas. Lie on your back and draw your knees towards your chest, wrapping your arms around your legs. Hold the pose while taking deep breaths, gently rocking side to side to massage the lower abdomen.

Marjaryasana-Bitilasana (Cat-Cow Pose). This dynamic combination of Cat and Cow poses helps massage the spine, stimulate digestion, and improve spinal flexibility. Begin on your hands and knees, with your wrists aligned under your shoulders and your knees under your hips. Inhale as you arch your back and lift your head and tailbone for Cow Pose, then exhale as you round your spine and tuck your chin for Cat Pose. Flow between these two poses with your breath for several rounds.

If you are someone like me who does not like heavy gym exercises then you can try these yoga poses or just take a walk in the garden. Taking walks can help to lighten the mood and keep the mind and body fresh. So, next time you feel stressed, just go for a good walk with your close one.

13

CHAPTER 13: KEEP GUT CLEAN

A clean and healthy gut is essential for overall well-being, as it plays a central role in digestion, nutrient absorption, and immune function. Maintaining a balanced and thriving gut ecosystem requires a holistic approach that encompasses dietary choices, lifestyle habits, and mindful practices. By implementing the following strategies, you can support digestive health, promote gut cleanliness, and optimize your overall health and vitality.

Dietary fiber acts as a natural cleanser for the digestive system, promoting regular bowel movements and sweeping waste and toxins out of the body. Incorporate a variety of fiber-rich foods into your diet, including fruits, vegetables, whole grains, legumes, nuts, and seeds. Aim for a diverse range of fiber sources to support gut microbiome diversity and health.

Adequate hydration is essential for maintaining gut motility and facilitating the elimination of waste products. Drink plenty of water throughout the day to keep the digestive system hydrated and functioning optimally. Herbal teas, infused water, and coconut water are also hydrating options that can support gut health.

Fermented foods are rich in probiotics, beneficial bacteria that support gut health and digestion. Incorporate fermented foods such as yogurt, kefir, sauerkraut, kimchi, tempeh, and miso into your diet regularly to promote a healthy balance of gut microbiota. These probiotic-rich foods help maintain gut cleanliness by crowding out harmful bacteria and supporting immune function.

Mindful eating involves paying attention to your food choices, chewing thoroughly, and savoring each bite. By slowing down and focusing on your meals, you can improve digestion, reduce overeating, and enhance nutrient absorption. Mindful eating also encourages awareness of hunger and fullness cues, helping prevent digestive discomfort and bloating.

Regular bowel movements are a key indicator of gut health and cleanliness. Strive for a consistent bowel movement pattern, aiming for at least one bowel movement per day. If you experience constipation or irregularity, incorporate additional fiber-rich foods, hydration, and physical activity into your routine to promote regularity.

Pay attention to how different foods and lifestyle habits affect your digestion and overall well-being. Notice any symptoms of digestive discomfort, bloating, or irregularity, and adjust your diet and lifestyle accordingly. Trust your body's signals and make choices that support gut health and cleanliness.

I always forget to take a poop break when I am busy completing my assignments. If you are someone who does that too then please take out five minutes to clean your gut. Also, keep drinking water. Cheers on cleaning your gut!!

14

BONUS: RECIPES FOR THE DAY YOU ARE FEELING SICK

Eating a proper diet on days when you are feeling sick is important. So, here are some sick day recipes. Give priority to the foods the doctor or physician has asked you to eat.

1. Gut-Healthy Green Smoothie:

Ingredients:

- 1 cup spinach or kale (fresh or frozen)
- 1/2 cup cucumber, chopped
- 1/2 cup pineapple chunks
- 1/2 banana
- 1 tablespoon chia seeds or ground flaxseeds
- 1 cup unsweetened almond milk or coconut water
- Optional: a squeeze of lemon juice or a knob of fresh ginger for added flavor

Instructions:

- Add all ingredients to a blender.
- Blend until smooth and creamy.
- Pour into a glass and enjoy as a refreshing breakfast or snack.

2. Quinoa Salad with Fermented Vegetables:
   Ingredients:

- 1 cup cooked quinoa, cooled
- 1/2 cup fermented vegetables (such as sauerkraut or kimchi), chopped
- 1/4 cup cucumber, diced
- 1/4 cup cherry tomatoes, halved
- 2 tablespoons fresh parsley, chopped
- 2 tablespoons extra-virgin olive oil
- 1 tablespoon apple cider vinegar
- Salt and pepper to taste

Instructions:

- In a large bowl, combine cooked quinoa, fermented vegetables, cucumber, cherry tomatoes, and parsley.
- In a small bowl, whisk together olive oil, apple cider vinegar, salt, and pepper to make the dressing.
- Pour the dressing over the salad and toss until well combined.
- Serve chilled or at room temperature as a nutritious side dish or light meal.

3. Ginger Turmeric Carrot Soup:
   Ingredients:

- 1 tablespoon coconut oil or olive oil
- 1 onion, diced
- 2 cloves garlic, minced
- 1 tablespoon fresh ginger, grated
- 1 teaspoon ground turmeric
- 4 large carrots, peeled and chopped
- 4 cups vegetable broth
- Salt and pepper to taste
- Fresh cilantro or parsley for garnish (optional)

Instructions:

1. Heat oil in a large pot over medium heat. Add diced onion and sauté until translucent.
2. Add minced garlic, grated ginger, and ground turmeric to the pot, and sauté for another minute until fragrant.
3. Add chopped carrots and vegetable broth to the pot. Bring to a boil, then reduce heat and simmer until carrots are tender, about 15-20 minutes.
4. Use an immersion blender to puree the soup until smooth. Alternatively, transfer the soup to a blender and blend until smooth (be careful when blending hot liquids).
5. Season with salt and pepper to taste.
6. Serve hot, garnished with fresh cilantro or parsley if desired. Enjoy this warming and nourishing soup for a comforting meal that supports gut health.

Hope you enjoy them. :) :)

15

CONCLUSION:

Firstly, I would like to thank you for reading my first ever book. I am so happy to complete it. I hope you enjoyed reading it. I would like to sincerely apologise for any mistake I did or if I made you feel hurt in any sense then I am really sorry. Being a beginner into writing I might have made many mistakes. Please don't take them seriously. With this I hope you have a healthy gut health.

Also, don't forget to drink that water. And I would appreciate it if you leave me a nice review on Amazon. Again, thanks a lot :)

Finally, cheers to you!!!!!!

16

REFERENCES

Kripalu Center for Yoga & Health. "Ayurvedic Wisdom for Better Digestion." Kripalu. Retrieved on May 27th, 2024. https://kripalu.org/resources/ayurvedic-wisdom-better-digestion#:~:text=Chew%20Your%20Food%20Properly&text=One%20of%20Ayurveda's%20golden%20eating,(which%20Ayurveda%20also%20recommends).

WebMD. "What Is Saliva?" WebMD. Retrieved on May 27th, 2024. https://www.webmd.com/oral-health/what-is-saliva

University of Chicago Medicine. "Specific Bacteria in the Small Intestine Are Crucial for Fat Absorption." University of Chicago Medicine. Retrieved on May 28th, 2024. https://www.uchicagomedicine.org/forefront/gastrointestinal-articles/2018/april/specific-bacteria-in-the-small-intestine-are-crucial-for-fat-absorption

Healthline. "Lactobacillus Acidophilus: Benefits, Side Effects, and More." Healthline. Retrieved on May 28th, 2024 from https://www.healthline.com/nutrition/lactobacillus-acidophilus#TOC_TITLE_HDR_

<u>3</u>

World Health Organization. "Obesity." World Health Organization. Retrieved on May 27th, 2024 from https://www.who.int/health-topics/obesity#tab=tab_1

ScienceDirect. "The Relationship between Sleep and Digestive Health." ScienceDirect. Retrieved on May 28th, 2024 from https://www.sciencedirect.com/science/article/pii/S075333222200066X

Medical News Today. "Why Do I Feel Sleepy After Eating?" Medical News Today. Retrieved on May 28th, 2024 from https://www.medicalnewstoday.com/articles/323379#:~:text=Feeling%20sleepy%20after%20eating%20can,especially%20tired%20after%20a%20meal.

Verywell Health. "Eating Before Bed: What to Avoid." Verywell Health. Retrieved on May 28th, 2024 from
https://www.verywellhealth.com/eating-before-bed-3014981#:~:text=As%20a%20general%20rule%20of,move%20into%20your%20small%20intestine.

Digestive Health Associates of Texas. "The Bittersweet Truth." Digestive Health Associates of Texas. Retrieved on May 28th, 2024 from https://dhat.com/gastroenterology-blog/the-bittersweet-truth

Mayo Clinic. "Digestion: How Long Does It Take?" Mayo Clinic. Retrieved on May 28th, 2024 from https://www.mayoclinic.org/healthy-lifestyle/nutrition-and-healthy-eating/expert-answers/digestion/faq-20058348#:~:text=In%20fact%2C%20drinking%20water%20during,softer%2C%20which%20helps%20prevent%20constipation.

Healthline. "The 3-Day Gut Reset Plan: Does It Work?" Healthline. Retrieved on May 28th, 2024 from https://www.healthline.com/health/digestive-health/3-day-gut-reset

BBC Good Food. "Gut-Friendly Recipes." BBC Good Food. Retrieved on May 28th, 2024 from https://www.bbcgoodfood.com/recipes/collection/gut-friendly-recipes

58

17

GRATITUDE

F irstly, Thanks for reading !!!!
I would like to thank everyone who believed in me and supported me till the very end.